Keto

Your Ultimate Guide to Low-Carb Friendly Options at America's Favorite Restaurants

By Jason Michaels

Table of Contents

Keto Diet on the Go:.. 1
Table of Contents... 2
Introduction.. 6
Chapter 1: Keto Options: Well-Known Chain Restaurants... 9
Chapter 2: Keto Options at Generic Non-Chain/Mom & Pop Restaurants... 81
Chapter 3: Keto Options at Convenience Stores & Gas Stations... 90
Chapter 4: Keto Options: Low Carb Alcoholic & Coffee Beverages... 95
Chapter 5: Keto Imposters &"Contraband"................ 100
Chapter 6: Helpful Tips & Guidelines......................... 106
Conclusion.. 114

© Copyright 2018 by Jason Michaels - All rights reserved.

The following eBook is reproduced below with the goal of providing information that is as accurate and reliable as possible. Regardless, purchasing this eBook can be seen as consent to the fact that both the publisher and the author of this book are in no way experts on the topics discussed within and that any recommendations or suggestions that are made herein are for entertainment purposes only. Professionals should be consulted as needed prior to undertaking any of the action endorsed herein.

This declaration is deemed fair and valid by both the American Bar Association and the Committee of Publishers Association and is legally binding throughout the United States.

Furthermore, the transmission, duplication or reproduction of any of the following work including specific information will be considered an illegal act irrespective of if it is done electronically or in print. This extends to creating a secondary or tertiary copy of the work or a recorded copy and is only allowed with express written consent from the Publisher. All additional right reserved.

The information in the following pages is broadly considered to be a truthful and accurate account of facts and as such any inattention, use or misuse of the information in question by the reader will render any resulting actions solely under their purview. There are no scenarios in which the publisher or the original author of this work can be in any fashion deemed liable for any hardship or damages that may befall them after undertaking information described herein.

Additionally, the information in the following pages is intended only for informational purposes and should thus be thought of as universal. As befitting its nature, it is presented without assurance regarding its prolonged validity or interim quality. Trademarks that are mentioned are done without written consent and can in no way be considered an endorsement from the trademark holder.

Introduction

You've conquered the first step by getting your body into ketosis. One of the many perks of this eating lifestyle is its sustainability. There are so many good foods that you can eat while in ketosis that will keep you satisfied and you won't even miss the bread! However, it's one thing to stick to the plan when you're doing your own meal prep. It's a whole new ballgame when you take your new eating habits out into the world. There are a few things you can do before reaching the restaurant of choice that will hopefully make the process a bit easier.

First, when possible, try not go out to eat on an empty stomach. If you're already somewhat satisfied you'll be able to resist temptations that much better. Even if you chug a glass of room temperature water before you leave, your stomach will feel more full.

If you've planned ahead, do your research before getting to the restaurant. Almost every chain restaurant has its full menu publically available. Decide which direction you want to take your meal and any off-menu modifications you might want to make. That way, when it comes time to order you'll know exactly what you want and how many carbs it will cost you.

Pack food ahead of time for trips. That will make you less likely to splurge on carby snacks at the gas station or airport.

Finally, don't stress out! It's understandable that asking for off-menu items can be a bit intimidating. There is always the risk that your dining companion might not understand or the order might arrive incorrect or incomplete. And that's okay! Because it will happen, on occasion, but at the end of the day, you are the one that matters.

So get ready to dive into the low-carb faction of the restaurant world. Bon appetit!

Side Note: net carbs are calculated by subtracting total fiber from total carbs

There are plenty of books on this subject on the market, thanks again for choosing this one! Every effort was made to ensure it is full of as much useful information as possible, please enjoy!

Chapter 1: Keto Options: Well-Known Chain Restaurants

Eating out, in general, can make it difficult to maintain dieting goals. Sticking to a diet at our favorite, well-known restaurants can up the challenge considerably. Thankfully, healthier trends in food preparation and low-carb options made available have made an appearance in a wide variety of our better-known chains.

Denny's

Good ol' Denny's; comforting, easy on the pocketbook, and they're always open! Resisting favorites could be difficult at this family favorite sit-down restaurant, but where there is a will, there is a way. And thankfully, there are quite a few ways to make these potentially carb-loaded meals much more keto friendly. Many of these low-carb options are appropriate for breakfast, lunch, or dinner.

T-Bone Steak & Eggs: This is about as perfect for low-carb eating as you can get...if all you were served was the steak and the eggs. Forgoing sides is a sacrifice that must be made, so to keep this favorite keto friendly, leave out extras such as toast and hash browns and it comes to about 1g net carbs.

Grand Slam (build-your-own): The Grand Slam is definitely on the favorites list. Here is a list of ingredients you could use to customize it to your liking and diet goals:

Bacon (2 strips= 1g net carbs), turkey bacon (2 strips= 1g net carbs), sausage (2 links= 0g net carbs), eggs (2= 1g net carbs), egg whites (2= 1g net carbs), grilled ham (3oz. slice= 3g net carbs), gouda-apple chicken sausage (1 link= 2g net carbs).

Use this list to mix and match to your liking, staying away from the pancakes, of course.

Favorite Omelettes: Denny's offers a variety of omelettes that are typically Keto friendly as they are, just be sure to leave out the "carby" sides:

Ham & Cheese Omelette: 7g net carbs

Ultimate Omelette®: 8g net carbs

Loaded Veggie Omelette: 7g net carbs

Philly Cheese-steak Omelette: 11g net carbs

Skillets: Denny's skillets are another great option, just be sure to get them without the potatoes. There was no data available on the exact net carbs on the skillets, but as long as they are potato free they should all fall below 10g:

Fit Fare® Veggie Skillet

Crazy Spicy Skillet (option to add eggs)

Supreme Skillet (option to add eggs)

Wild Alaska Salmon Skillet

Santa Fe Skillet (option to add eggs)

Salads & Sides: You can never go wrong with a salad! Well, I guess technically you can, but as long as you stick to these low-carb options you'll be on the right track:

Prime Rib Cobb Salad (no dressing): 12g net carbs

Veggies with Ranch Dip: 3g net carbs

Avocado Chicken Caesar Salad (16 oz.): 8g net carbs

Tilapia Ranchero (no bread): 3g net carbs

T-Bone Steak (no bread): 5g net carbs

Sirloin Steak (no bread): 3g net carbs

Burgers/Sandwiches: None of these options will start as low-carb because of the bread and some of the condiments. To make these sandwiches keto friendly, order without the bread, possibly in a lettuce wrap, avoid sugary condiments such as BBQ sauce and ketchup, and skip the fries or substitute with cut veggies. Try to limit or avoid fruit as sides.

Condiments: Condiment options will probably be very similar across the board at any restaurant, but here are some specific to Denny's:

Ranch Dressing (1.5oz): 1g net carbs

Buffalo Sauce (2oz): 2g net carbs

Blue Cheese Dressing (1.5oz): 3g net carbs

Caesar Dressing (1.5oz): 0g net carbs

Italian Dressing (Fat free, 1.5oz): 4g net carbs

Sour Cream (1.5oz): 2g net carbs

IHOP

IHOP options will be very similar to Denny's and the same rules for entrees, sandwiches and burgers will apply: skip the bread, potatoes, and sweet condiments. Some of the main menu, however, can be ordered with little to no alterations.

Omelettes: Something to keep in mind; some of the research has discovered that IHOP puts pancake batter in their eggs when they make the omelettes, which obviously has an effect on the net carbs. Be sure to request real eggs when ordering.

Colorado Omelette: 13g net carbs

Avocado, Bacon, Cheese Omelette: 5g net carbs

Corned Beef Hash & Cheese Omelette: 20g net carbs

Bacon Temptation Omelette: 10g net carbs

Bacon, Sausage, and Eggs: When in doubt, keep it simple...good ol' bacon and eggs! Eggs (basic serving size is usually 2) can be fried, poached, scrambled, or boiled and they will contain about 1-2g net carbs. Sausage or bacon are usually about 1g net carbs for an order. Order just bacon and/or sausage and eggs (no sides) and you'll have a fulfilling meal that will keep you in ketosis.

Salads/Dressings: As with any salad, the danger is most often in the dressing, both the type and the quantity.

Grilled Chicken Cobb: 10g net carbs (without the dressing)

House Salad: 3g net carbs (without the dressing)

Caesar Salad (side, 12g net carbs, without the dressing)

The dressings are what launch the net carbs upward, so take care when ordering! Get the dressing on the side to help keep the carb load down.

Waffle House

Yet another diner style, comforting, carb-laden restaurant. And still, there are plenty of low carb options to choose from.

Omelettes: Avoid sides (toast, hash browns, etc.).

Ham & Cheese Omelette: 10g net carbs

Fiesta Omelette: 7g net carbs

Cheese-steak Omelette: 6g net carbs

Breakfast Staples

Bacon (3 slices): 0g net carbs

Country Ham (1 slice): 0g net carbs

Sausage (2 patties): 0g net carbs

Eggs w/ Cheese (2 eggs, equivalent of 1 slice of cheese): 1g net carbs

Sausage Egg & Cheese Wrap: 25g Net Carbs

Meat: Most meat choices, without any kind of sauce or gravy, are going to be 0g net carbs.

Burgers/Sandwiches: Same rule applies as before; skip the bread, sweet condiments, and fries. Maybe try adding a fried egg on top of a bunless burger to make it more interesting.

California Pizza Kitchen

In order to stay low carb at California Pizza Kitchen, you may have to forgo the pizza. However, their low carb options are still very good and will provide a fulfilling meal while remaining in ketosis.

Salads

Italian Chopped Salad (half portion): 9g net carbs

Classic Caesar Salad (full portion): 12g net carbs

Roasted Veggie & Grilled Shrimp Salad (half portion): 17g net carbs

California Cobb Salad (full portion, including ranch dressing): 13g net carbs

Appetizers/Entrees

Lettuce Wraps (order with chicken or shrimp or both!)

Grilled Chicken Chimichurri: 13g net carbs

Fire-Roasted Chile Relleno: 20g net carbs

Grilled Chicken Breast (no sauces/sides): 0g net carbs

Power Bowls: These are definitely healthier options; for keto diets, they may still need to be tweaked just a bit. No net carb info available, but here are some suggestions to make sure these bowls stay keto friendly:

Shanghai Power Bowl: This meal comes with shrimp and a variety of vegetables such as cauliflower, baby broccoli, carrots, and zucchini. It also includes Forbidden Rice® and house made Shanghai sauce, both of which should probably be held off (or at least on the side) to keep the carbs down.

Santa Fe Bowl: This bowl includes lime chicken, sweet corn, tomatoes, black beans, avocado, poblano peppers, red cabbage, and toasted pepitas on top of spinach and cilantro farr0. It is served with CPK's house made ranch. To keep this bowl keto friendly, it would be best to skip the corn and ask for dressing on the side.

Banh Mi Bowl: This bowl consists of baby kale, quinoa, mint, and cilantro topped by grilled chicken, radishes, watermelon, avocado, carrots, bean sprouts, cucumbers, scallions, and sesame seeds. It comes with CPK's chili and lime vinaigrette and Serrano peppers. While quinoa is very healthy, it is also very high in protein. Unused protein is broken down into sugar and stored as fat.

Cauliflower Crust: CPK has recently come out with a cauliflower crust, reportedly consisting of cauliflower, rice flour, mozzarella, and some spices and herbs. This is great news for vegetarians but perhaps not so much for keto and low-carb as one slice is 90 calories and has 14g net carbs. It might be best to stick with non-pizza meals in order to remain in ketosis.

Chili's

Chili's actually has a section in their menu called "Guiltless Grills". Some items on this part of the menu may be a bit too high in starch, which bumps net carbs up to 50g and over. However, there are a few specific dishes that are perfect for the keto diet (all listed not including the sides that come with some of the entrees).

Guiltless Grills & Other Main Dishes

Guiltless Cedar Plank Tilapia: Seasoned tilapia fillet with Chili's house made pico de gallo and served on a cedar plank; 3g net carbs.

Guiltless Grilled Salmon: 8oz of salmon seasoned and seared; 5g net carbs.

Salmon with Garlic and Herbs: 1g net carbs

Guiltless Carne Asada Steak Sirloin: The meat is seasoned and flame grilled and also comes with the house made pico de gallo; 5g net carbs.

Spicy Garlic & Lime Grilled Shrimp: 7g net carbs

Pepper Pals Grilled Chicken Platter (on the kids' menu): 4g net carbs

Chili's Classic Sirloins: 1g net carbs

Starters

Caesar Salad (side portion, no croutons!): approximately 6g net carbs

Triple Dipper Wings over Buffalo with Blue Cheese: 2g net carbs

Cup Chicken Enchilada: 8g net carbs

Terlinga Chili (cup): 7g net carbs

Lunch Combo House Salad (Hold the dressing): 9g net carbs

Extras/Sides

Dressings: Blue Cheese, Avocado Ranch, and Caesar

Avocado Slices

Side of Guacamole (small)

Sautéed Mushrooms

All Cheeses

Sour Cream

Steamed Broccoli

Cut veggies (celery, carrots)

Applebee's

Applebee's also has a low carb section on their menu, making it much easier to pick keto friendly meals.

Starters

Double Crunch Bone-In Wings (either with blue cheese or ranch dressing): 13g net carbs

Double Crunch Bone-In Wings (no sauce or dressing): 10g net carbs

Double Crunch Bone-In Wings (classic Buffalo): 13g net carbs

Main Dishes (from the grill)

Doubled-Glazed Baby Back Ribs (both half rack and full rack, no sauce): 0g net carbs

Fire-Grilled Shrimp Skewer: 1g net carbs

12oz Top Sirloin (Butcher's Reserve): 0g net carbs

USDA Top Sirloin 6oz: 1g net carbs

USDA Top Sirloin 8oz: 2g net carbs

Shrimp 'N Parmesan Sirloin: 5g net carbs

Grilled Chicken Breast: 0g net carbs

Lunch Dishes

Thai Shrimp Salad: 12g net carbs

Tomato Basil Soup (cup): 13g net carbs

Southwest Black Bean Soup (cup): 12g net carbs

Grilled Chicken Caesar Salad (no croutons!): 8g net carbs

House Salads: Some of these salads are a bit higher in the carb range than you might want, especially if you plan on getting an entrée as well. Be mindful of dressing choice/quantity and leave off extras such as croutons, chips, fruit, and nuts.

House Salad w/ Buttermilk Ranch: 13g net carbs
House Salad w/ Garlic Caesar: 13g net carbs

House Salad w/ Blue Cheese: 13g net carbs

House Salad w/ Lemon Olive Oil Vinaigrette: 10g net carbs

House Salad w/ Mexi Ranch: 13g net carbs

House Salad w/ Italian: 15g net carbs

House Salad w/ Green Goddess: 12g net carbs

Small Caesar: 9g net carbs

Green Goddess Wedge Salad: 9g net carbs

House Salad (no dressing): 10g net carbs

Sides

Garlicky Green Beans w/ Bacon: 7g net carbs

Fire-Grilled Veggies: 6g net carbs

Steamed Broccoli: 3g net carbs

Wendy's

As with other restaurants serving burger and sandwiches, all of these low-carb options from Wendy's are bunless.

Burger & Meat Options (no condiments or toppings)

Jr. Hamburger Patty: 0g net carbs

Single Hamburger Patty: 0g net carbs

Grilled Chicken Breast: 3g net carbs

Applewood Smoked Bacon (1 strip): 0g net carbs

Toppings/Condiments: The stand-alone meat options are very low in net carbs. Which means you can add to your order as you keep track of the carb count in these condiments and toppings.

Cheeses: American 1 slice= 1g net carbs, Asiago 1 slice= 1g net carbs, cheddar 1 slice= 0g net carbs, shredded cheddar= 1g net carbs, cheddar cheese sauce= 1g net carbs

Mayonnaise: 0g net carbs

Mustard: 0g net carbs

Pickles, onions, and iceberg lettuce: all 0g net carbs

Tomato: 1 slice= 1g net carbs

Tartar Sauce: 0g net carbs

Salads

Garden Salad (without dressing and croutons): 5g net carbs

Caesar Salad (without dressing and croutons): 4g net carbs

Sauces/Dressing

Ranch: 2g net carbs

Buttermilk Ranch (dipping sauce): 2g net carbs

Light Ranch: 2g net carbs

Italian: 4g net carbs

Lemon Garlic Caesar: 2g net carbs

Thousand Island: 5g net carbs

Meal Pairing Ideas: Now that we know individual options, we can mix and match meals. These won't necessarily have a spot on the actual menu, but they d0 fulfill the requirements for low-carb options.

Three Double-Stack Cheeseburgers (dry, no bun) with pickles, wrapped in lettuce: 3g net carbs

Grilled Chicken (dry, no bun), garden side salad w/ ranch, Diet Coke: 7g net carbs

Two Jr. Bacon Cheeseburgers (dry, no bun) with Caesar salad (no dressing or croutons), and small Minute Maid Lemonade: 11g net carbs

Triple Baconator (dry, no bun) mayo on the side, bottle of water: 3g net carbs

KFC

Everything about KFC says "comfort food". There is nothing specifically on the menu labeled as low-carb, but if KFC is absolutely the last option for a meal, there is a smart way to order to stay on the keto diet.

Meal Ideas

There aren't a lot of chicken options that will stick with the keto diet, so the Kentucky Grilled Chicken Breast is probably the only way to go:

Two Kentucky Grilled Chicken Breasts with a small side of green beans and maybe a side of creamy buffalo dip comes to about 6g net carbs.

Sides

Caesar Salad (no dressing): 1g net carbs

Side Salad (no dressing): 1g net carbs

Sauce

Creamy Buffalo: 2g net carbs

Buttermilk Ranch: 2g net carbs

Dressing

Marzetti Light Italian: 2g net carbs

KFC Creamy Parmesan Caesar: 4g net carbs

Heinz Buttermilk Ranch: 1g net carbs

McDonald's

All of the McDonald's low-carb options take out the bun or bread (biscuit, muffins) and have no ketchup included. The buns alone on the burgers account for more than ¾ of the carb count listed on the nutrition facts!

Breakfast: There really aren't a whole lot of low-carb options for breakfast since most of their famous breakfast options include muffins, biscuits, and/or syrup.

Modified Egg McMuffin: take out the muffin, keep the egg, American cheese, and ham or sausage and it goes from about 30g net carbs to 2.
Basically, any other item on the breakfast menu would follow the same rules: take out bread and sauces and stay away from the hash browns!

Burgers/Sandwiches: Again, follow these simple rules: no bread or condiments (except for mustard), get them wrapped in lettuce instead. All the meats (as long as they're dry) have 0g net carbs and almost all of the toppings have 0-1g net carbs. Absolutely no fries!

Some good low carb options are:

Big Mac (dry no buns): 6g net carbs

Quarter Pounder w/ Cheese (dry, no buns): 7g net carbs

Bacon Clubhouse Burger (dry, no buns): 8g net carbs

Grilled Chicken (dry, no bun): 2g net carbs

Filet-o-Fish (dry, no bun): splurge w/ cheese a side of tartar sauce comes to about 10g net carbs

Salads

Side Salads (no dressing): 2g net carbs

Caesar w/ Grilled Chicken (no croutons): 9g net carbs

Bacon Ranch w/ Grilled Chicken: 6g net carbs

Dressing Packets

Creamy Caesar: 4g net carbs

Low Fat Balsamic Vinaigrette: 6g net carbs

Ranch: 2-4g net carbs

Taco Bell

Taco Bell doesn't have a specifically low-carb menu either, but here are some options for making some of the regular menu items keto friendly. If you're stressing and feel like you just can't find anything, simply removing beans, potatoes, and rice from dishes will dramatically reduce carbs. All hot sauces are 0g net carbs.

Breakfast

Mini Skillet Bowl- with eggs, pico de gallo and nacho cheese (hold the potatoes): 3g net carbs

Power Menu Bowls

Steak Power Bowl (hold beans and rice): 1g net carbs

Ground Beef Power Bowl (hold beans and rice): 7g net carbs

Chicken Power Bowl (hold beans and rice): 5g net carbs

Add-Ons (all 0-2g net carbs)

Steak: 1g net carb

Fire Grilled Chicken: 0g net carbs

Shredded Chicken: 1g net carbs

Seasoned Ground Beef: 1g net carbs

Guacamole: 1,5g net carbs

Bacon: 0g net carbs

Shredded Cheddar: 0g net carbs

Sausage Crumbles: 0g net carbs

Shredded 3 Cheese Blend: 0g net carbs

Sour Cream: 2g net carbs

Extra Cheese Sauce: 2g net carbs

Jalapenos: 0.5g net carbs

Chipotle

Chipotle is a little more health/low-carb friendly than some of the other fast food choices without technically having the options on the menu. They make an effort to keep their ingredients fresh and just about anything on their menu can be made as a salad, which is going to be the best keto option.

For the salad bowls, you can get any of the meats (steak, chicken, pork, barbacoa), cheese, sour cream (make sure it's full fat), red salsa, and guacamole. Steer clear of corn and the green salsas and mix and match all you want!

Sizzler

The buffet side of Sizzler is potentially very dangerous for a keto diet even though it's just a salad bar. There are some very good choices on their menus for keto entrees, but you will have to be careful with the salad bar.

Salads

Asian Chopped Salad (1/2 cup): 3g net carbs

Cucumber Tomato Salad (1/2 cup): 4g net carbs

Greek Salad (1/2 cup): 1g net carbs

Main Dishes

Grilled Salmon w/ Vegetable Medley (6oz, no tartar sauce): 10g net carbs

Italian Herbed Chicken w/ Steamed Broccoli: 9g net carbs

Hibachi Chicken w/ Steamed Broccoli: 12g net carbs (Note: get without sauces and pineapple to bring carb count down)

Shrimp Skewers w/ Cilantro Rice & Steamed Broccoli: 33g net carbs (Note: this is a pretty high carb count! Asking for no rice will bring it down considerably, also request no garlic margarine.)

South Atlantic Red Shrimp Skewers w/ Steamed Broccoli: 42g net carbs (Note: this dish also comes with cilantro rice; no rice will bring carb count down.)

Shrimp Skewers w/ Cilantro Rice and Vegetable Medley: 34g net carbs (Note: another higher carb dish; get it without rice and garlic margarine.)

Tri Tip Steak w/ Vegetable Medley (6oz steak): 8g net carbs

Sides

Tri-Color Quinoa Kale Salad: 13g net carbs (Note: Quinoa is high in protein; if you choose this, make sure you are monitoring protein intake for the rest of the day.)

Steamed Broccoli: 7g net carbs

Vegetable Medley: 8g net carbs

Subway

Obviously, sandwiches are out! But thankfully Subway will make most of their sandwiches as salads that can be tweaked to make them more filling and with the right amount of fat. You can add veggies, usually with no extra charge, or ask for double the meat. You will most likely have to pay for that, but it will make the salads more filling.

Chopped Tuna Salad w/ oil & vinegar (get with extra bacon!): 2g net carbs

Spicy Italian Chopped Salad: 5g net carbs

Cold Cut Combo Salad: 5g net carbs

Subway Club Salad w/ oil & vinegar (double the meat): 5g net carbs

Italian BMT Salad (double the meat): 5g net carbs

Roasted Chicken Patty Salad w/ oil & vinegar: 3g net carbs

Red Robin

If it's burgers you want, the easiest way to keep it Keto is to skip the bun and wrap them in lettuce. Forgo most sauces and condiments or ask for them on the side. You can add bacon for 0g net carbs or cheese for only 1g net carbs.

Wedgie Burger: Red Robin actually does have a specifically low-carb meal on their menu and it's called the Wedgie Burger. It comes on a lettuce wedge and includes bacon, guacamole, tomato, and onion. If you don't want the beef patty you can substitute it with a chicken or turkey burger.

Bottomless Salad: Red Robin is famous for their bottomless fries and thankfully you can swap the fries out for bottomless salad.

Wedge Salad: Their wedge salad is constructed the same way as the Wedgie Burger, just without the burger meat. It is a wedge of iceberg lettuce topped with blue cheese, tomatoes, bacon bits, and onion straws. Skip the onions to make it keto appropriate.

Golden Corral

Buffet style restaurants could make it more difficult to be disciplined. One of the upsides, however, is the fact that you get to fill your own plate. You don't have to feel like you're inconveniencing the servers and chefs. Here are some low-carb meal ideas from Golden Corral. Keep in mind: according to their nutrition facts, quite a few of their dishes contain wheat and soy.

Breakfast: There are not an abundance of keto friendly breakfasts at Golden Corral, but they do have some low-carb breakfast staples you can mix and match to create a meal.

Bacon: 3 pieces= 0g net carbs

Chorizo & Eggs: ½ cup serving= 2g net carbs

Made-To-Order Eggs: 1 egg= 1g net carbs

Sausage: 1 link= 1g net carbs

Meat Dishes: Golden Corral has countless meats prepared in a variety of different ways. Not all of them are keto friendly due to how they're prepared. Here are a few that are good for low-carb diets that don't contain wheat and/or soy.

Garlic Herb Butter Sirloin: 3oz= 1g net carbs

Garlic Parmesan Sirloin: 3oz= 1g net carbs

Lemon Rosemary Sirloin: 3oz= 1g net carbs

Rib Eye: 3oz= 0g net carbs

Boneless Chicken Wings w/ Frank's Hot Sauce: 3 pieces= 0g net carbs

Rotisserie Chicken: 1 piece= 1g net carbs

Baby Back Pork Ribs: 1 rib= 3g net carbs

BBQ Pork: 3oz= 4g net carbs

Grilled Ham Steaks: 2 pieces= 5g net carbs

Seafood: All the seafood dishes contain soy and wheat; it would best to steer clear of those.

Sides: All of the sides either contain wheat and soy or are too high in carbs to be keto friendly.

Vegetables

Steamed Broccoli: ½ cup= 3g net carbs

Steamed Cauliflower: ½ cup= 1g net carbs

Sautéed Spinach: ½ cup= 1g net carbs

Vegetable Trio: ½ cup= 4g net carbs

Dairy Queen

Obviously, the ice cream is off limits. But some of the regular menu favorites can be modified into low-carb options.

Turkey BLT (without ciabatta roll): Sliced turkey, melted Swiss cheese, bacon, lettuce, tomato, and mayo. Hold off on the mayo to bring carbs down even more: 3g net carbs

Original Cheeseburger (without the bun): Beef patty, lettuce, American cheese, pickles, onions and mustard. Only add mayo if you need the extra fat: 3g net carbs

Grilled Chicken BLT Salad: Bacon, chicken, cheese, lettuce, and ranch dressing: without dressing= 7g net carbs, with dressing= 10g net carbs

FlameThrower GrillBurger (without the bun, spicy!): Either one half pound patty or (depending on location) two quarter pound patties, creamy jalapeno sauce, jalapeno bacon, lettuce, sliced jalapeños, tomato, and pepper jack: 4g net carbs

Chicken Bacon Ranch (without ciabatta roll): Chicken breasts, tomato, lettuce, melted Swiss, ranch, and bacon: 5g net carbs

Starbucks (Food Only)

Starbucks has developed a good balance of keeping classic food selections and bringing in new ones. They seem to have focused more on low or reduced fat options, but there are a couple of things that can be eaten on a keto diet. Note: "reduced fat" items are *not* keto options.

Breakfast

Sous Vide Egg Bites: Rich and yummy, these are technically keto friendly but they are on the high end of the carb spectrum, so keep track of carb intake the rest of the day: 9g net carbs per order

Snacks

Snack Boxes: the protein box does include a hard-boiled egg and some cheese, but the rest of the contents aren't keto friendly.

Kind Bars: These are keto friendly, but they are also high in carbs (8g) and they're not even a full meal.

Wingstop

Chicken is definitely a must have for keto diets, but not all forms are healthy. Here are some wing options at Wingstop that are keto friendly. Note: the info listed below is based on an order of 10 wings.

Plain Wings: 0g net carbs

Atomic: 5g net carbs

Mild: 0g net carbs

Garlic Parmesan: 0g net carbs

Cajon: 0g net carbs

Original (hot!): 0g net carbs

Louisiana Rub: 0g net carbs

Lemon Pepper: 0g net carbs

Pair the wings with ranch or blue cheese and celery sticks!

Cheesecake Factory

This chain is absolutely a family favorite! Most of the menu, unfortunately, is not keto friendly but there are a few meals that fit the carb requirements.

Starters: Almost all of the starters are upwards of 30g net carbs and more. The carpaccio is the one option that might have a low enough carb count to work: 11g net carbs (serves 2).

Salads (small options)

Boston House Salad: 11g net carbs

BLT Salad: 15g net carbs

Caesar Salad (with or without chicken): Less than 20g net carbs

Cobb Salad (lunch side): Less than 20g net carbs

Entrees (will have to be modified)

Sandwiches and burgers: order them dry, without the bun/bread

Steak, Seafood, Sides

One option outside of modifying meals on your own is taking advantage of Cheesecake Factory's make-your-own meals. Choose as low carb meats and sides as you can.

Steak Diane: 10g net carbs

Petite Rib Eye: 24g net carbs

Petite Fillet: 23g net carbs

Grilled Salmon: 3g net carbs

Grilled Tuna: 3g net carbs

Grilled Mahi Mahi: 3g net carbs

Herb-Crusted Salmon: 8g net carbs

Green Beans (side): 6g net carbs

Sautéed Spinach (side): 6g net carbs

Asparagus (side): 7g net carbs

Broccoli (side): 9g net carbs

Olive Garden

Italian restaurants can be daunting for any dieter, and there really aren't many low-carb options available. But they do have a few and they even have their own spot on the menu.

Salads & Sides:

Fresh Spinach Salad: 3g net carbs

Oven Roasted Asparagus: 1g net carbs

Bottomless Salad: essentially everything in this salad is keto friendly; even the dressing, up to a certain amount. If you're going that route, ask for a cup of dressing on the side.

Entrees

Herb Grilled Salmon & Broccoli: 1g net carbs

Steak Toscano & Grilled Vegetables: 32g net carbs

Mixed Grill Steak & Chicken Skewers with Grilled Vegetables: 20g net carbs

Alfredo sauce is actually fairly low carb so you can order a side of that for your veggies if you need to make the meal more interesting.

Five Guys Burgers

Five Guys has actually gone out of their way to make their menu low-carb optional, which definitely makes them stand out from the average fast food place. You can literally get any burger on the menu either bunless or in a tin salad-style. You can get the works, all of which are acceptable, except for the ketchup and maybe the mayo unless you need the fat. Here are just a few of the options Five Guys offers. The milkshakes are off limits!

Bunless Hot Dog in a Tin: with relish, onions, and mustard: 7g net carbs

Cheeseburger in a Lettuce Wrap: 1g net carbs

Bunless Bacon Double Cheeseburger in a Tin: try it with jalapeños, bacon, and cheese: 2g net carbs

In-N-Out

In-N-Out has also made an effort to offer low carb choices. They have an entire hidden menu; not all of them are low-carb but a few of them are. Ask for any of the burger protein style to skip the bun and get them wrapped in lettuce.

Double Double Protein Style: two patties, two slices of cheese, special sauce, and all the toppings: 8g net carbs

Cheeseburger Protein Style: single patty, single cheese, special sauce, and all the toppings: 8g net carbs

Hamburger Animal and Protein Style (secret menu): all the burgers can be ordered animal style; it just means the burger is fried in mustard and then they add grilled onions, more pickles, and extra special sauce: 11g net carbs

4x4 Cheeseburger Protein Style (secret menu): four patties, four slices of cheese, two slices of tomato, special sauce: 8g net carbs

3x3 Cheeseburger Protein Style (secret menu): exactly the same as the "quad" but with one less patty, etc.: 8g net carbs

Panera

Although Panera specializes in bread, pastries, and sandwiches, much of their menu can simply be ordered without the bread. They also have a selection of soups and salads that can be keto friendly.

Breakfast: Basically any of their breakfast sandwiches can be ordered without the bread and still function as a satisfying meal.

Ham, Egg, & Cheese Sandwich (without bread): 3g net carbs

Turkey Sausage, Egg White, & Spinach Sandwich (without bread): 2g net carbs

Sausage, Egg, & Cheese Sandwich (without the bread): 3g net carbs

Steak, Egg, & Cheese Bagel Sandwich (without the bagel): 3g net carbs

Lunch & Dinner

Steak & Baby Arugula Sandwich (on lettuce): 10g net carbs

Caesar Chicken Salad (without croutons): 6g net carbs

Green Goddess Cobb Salad (add chicken): 10g net carbs

Italian Sandwich (without bread): ham, sopressa, salami, arugula, provolone, giardiniera, and basil mayo (get the mayo on the side): 4g net carbs

Steak & White Cheddar (without bread): on a bed of lettuce: 7g net carbs

Roasted Turkey & Avocado BLT (without bread): 2g net carbs

Whataburger

Whataburger is yet another burger chain with a menu that can be easily modified into low-carb meals. Here are just a few examples of how to make these burgers keto friendly.

Breakfast

Sausage, Egg, & Cheese Sandwich (without bun): 0g net carbs

Scrambled Eggs & Bacon (3 slices of bacon): 3g net carbs

Sausage, Egg, & Cheese Taquito (no tortilla): 3g net carbs

Lunch & Dinner

Double Meat Whataburger add Double Cheese, Bacon, & Jalapeno (without the bun): 5g net carbs (add a side of ranch for about 1 additional g of net carbs)

Grilled Chicken Melt w/ Lettuce (without the bun): 3g net carbs

Whataburger Patty Melt (without the bun): 2g net carbs

Garden Salad w/ Whatachik'n: 17g net carbs- to reduce carb count, get without the fried chicken and take off tomatoes and carrots. Ranch dressing adds about 1g additional net carb.

Cracker Barrel

This restaurant will forever be a family favorite with its great vibe and scrumptious down home meals. Cracker Barrel has also added some great low carb option to their menu.

Breakfast

Country Grilled Sampler: bacon, sausage, sliced tomatoes, and country ham: 4g net carbs (no toast, drop the tomatoes to lower carb count if needed)

Double Meat Breakfast: three eggs, sausage, bacon, and sliced tomatoes (no toast, drop tomatoes if needed).

Eggs 'n Meat: three eggs, sausage or bacon, and sliced tomatoes: 2 net carbs (no toast, drop tomatoes if needed).

Lunch or Dinner

Grilled Steak Salad: 7g net carbs (not including dressing)

Lemon Pepper Grilled Trout: 0g net carbs (not counting sides)

Half Pound Bacon Cheeseburger (no bun): 3g net carbs (not counting sides)

Grilled Roast Beef: 4g net carbs (not counting sides)

Sides

Blue Cheese Dressing: 2g net carbs

Buttermilk Ranch: 1g net carbs

Spicy Pork Rinds: 1g net carbs

Green Beans: 2g net carbs

Texas Roadhouse

Texas Roadhouse is a very popular steakhouse. Thankfully, with these types of restaurants, the options to order low-carb are fairly plentiful. Between the numerous steak dishes and their choice of salads, staying in ketosis should be a cinch at this restaurant.

Starters

Boneless Buffalo Wings (Hot Sauce): 8g net carbs

Boneless Buffalo Wings (Mild Sauce): 8g net carbs

Texas Red Chili (cup): 7g net carbs
Note: the bowl is considerably higher in carbs; if you are planning on eating an entrée as well, the cup would be the best option.

Salads

California Chicken Salad (meal size): 12g net carbs

Chicken Caesar (meal size, with dressing): 16g net carbs

Grilled Chicken (meal size): 13g net carbs

Grilled Salmon (meal size): 11g net carbs

Caesar (side): 9g net carbs

House Salad (side): 7g net carbs

Dressings

Blue Cheese (2oz): 4g net carbs

Ranch (2oz): 4g net carbs

Caesar (2oz): 4g net carbs

Steak Options (10g and under)

Dallas Filet (6oz): 4g net carbs

Dallas Filet (8oz): 6g net carbs

Ft. Worth Ribeye (10oz, 12oz, 16oz): 0g net carbs

New York/Kansas City Strip (8oz, 12oz): 1g net carbs

Prime Rib (10oz, 12oz): 5g net carbs

Chicken Options (10g and under)

Oven Roasted Half Chicken: 7g net carbs

Portobello Mushroom Chicken: 7g net carbs

Country Dinners (Pork)

Grilled Pork Chops (single): 3g net carbs

Grilled Pork Chops (double): 6g net carbs

Fish

Grilled Salmon (5oz, 8oz): 1g net carbs

Sides

Fresh Vegetables: 7g net carbs

Sautéed Mushrooms: 4g net carbs

Green Beans: 11g net carbs

Red Lobster

Seafood is fairly versatile as well. Many of the dishes are paired with butter sauces, which should be keto friendly. And they have a handy low-carb section on their menu to make ordering easy. And, as heart breaking as it is, you'll have to forgo the classic, addicting cheddar biscuits.

Starters

Buffalo Chicken Wings: 4g net carbs

Shellfish Dishes

Shrimp Your Way (Scampi): 3g net carbs

Wild-Caught Snow Crab Legs: 0g net carbs

Live Maine Lobster (1.25lb, steamed): 0g net carbs

Feasts & Combos

CYO-Garlic Shrimp Scampi: 3g net carbs

CYO- Fresh Wood-Grilled Tilapia: 1g net carbs

CYO- Wood Grilled Sea Scallops: 4g net carbs

CYO- 7oz Wood-Grilled Sirloin: 1g net carbs

Other Fish Dishes

Salmon New Orleans (half or full): 8g net carbs

Wild-Caught Flounder (oven broiled): 1g net carbs

Sides & Salads (under 10g net carbs)

Garden Salad: 9g net carbs

Fresh Asparagus: 2g net carbs

Grilled Shrimp (add to salad): 0g net carbs

Fresh Broccoli: 5g net carbs

Classic Lunch Dishes

Farm-Raised Blackened Catfish: 2g net carbs

Chapter 2: Keto Options at Generic Non-Chain/Mom & Pop Restaurants

Some of the best meals we've ever had have come from quaint little "mom & and pop" restaurants, many of them offering a variety of ethnic foods. They may not be big chain franchises but they make up for it with nostalgia and good food. One of the negatives of these dining establishments is that nutrition details will probably be much harder to come by. There are still plenty of options for making meals low-carb, they just won't be as easily accessible on the menu. If you find you are having trouble putting together a low-carb meal, it's never wrong to politely ask an establishment how some of their menu items are prepared. Here are some tips on how to make some of these ethnic and generic restaurant foods more keto friendly.

Italian

Whenever we think "Italian food", we immediately imagine pasta, bread, pizza, cheese, more bread...so, essentially, carb heaven! Italian food is easily a favorite for many people, and initially, it may seem that low-carb choices will be impossible to find. Thankfully, that is not the case.

Pasta and pizza are very much staples in Italian food restaurants here in America and a big part of these dishes are the toppings, which usually consist of good meats and healthy veggies. Try ordering a pasta or pizza meal but ask for the toppings to go over lettuce. If you can, make sure the vegetables are cooked in olive oil, or even butter, if it's full fat. Grass fed is preferable but not always attainable. Opt for straight olive oil and vinegar for the dressing, unless you've confirmed that their ranch or Caesar does not have excess amounts of sugar, especially if it's house-made.

Grilled chicken, beef, or fish will also most likely be on the menu, you'll just have to forgo carb-loaded sides and sauces. Pesto is an option to spread over chicken but use sparingly because of the pine nuts.

Antipasto ("before meal") platters are often available for appetizers. These plates usually consist of meats, vegetables, and sometimes seafood, all of which are excellent low-carb options.

Soups can be a good keto meal as well, as long as they are made with thinner broths rather than thicker "chowder" bases. Chowders often need starch and/or flour to make them thicken which will knock you out of ketosis very quickly. Steer clear of soups with pasta, beans, or gnocchi in them as well.

Mexican

Mexican cuisine is delicious and exciting, but much of it includes beans and rice in a variety of forms witch is not conducive to staying in ketosis. Requesting meals without the rice and beans will immediately lower the carb count.

You can get just about any meal that comes in a tortilla either on the side or over a bed of shredded lettuce. Cheese, full fat sour cream, red salsas, and avocado are all keto approved. Watch out for the additives in guacamole. If you would rather have that over plain avocado slices, be sure to ask what the ingredients are.

Any meat that is grilled is fine and you can even request it over fajita-grilled vegetables rather than inside of a tortilla. Sides such as ceviche and pico de gallo are also options for spicing up your modified meal.

Japanese/Sushi

A lot of Japanese and sushi dishes already cater to low-carb diets with little to no modification. Granted, sushi does come with rice so sashimi is a better choice. Avoid edamame as well; ½ a cup of those little guys easily reaches 9-10g net carbs!

Miso soup is a good low-carb choice. It is a good keto friendly starter and will help fill you up if you find you have limited keto options. Some Japanese restaurants have a dish called Konjac Ramen, which is one of the few noodle-type dishes that will be low-carb enough for your diet. The noodles are made out of the root of the elephant yam and the single serving size only comes to about 2-3g net carbs. Granted, there are other toppings on ramen bowls, so you will have to be conscientious about the other ingredients to keep it low carb.

As with the other restaurants, grilled meats are always a good choice provided they are not covered in any kind of sauce. Non-seafood options at sushi restaurants often consist of either beef or chicken teriyaki bowls. You could modify these by getting the sauce on the side and forgoing the rice.

Indian

Indian cuisine might be a bit more difficult to get low-carb options for. While the spices are very good, many of the dishes come with sauces and unless you're making it yourself, it could be difficult to find any without sugars or flours used to thicken them. Try to order meat dishes, with little to no sauce if possible, and always skip the naan and rice.

Tandoori chicken can be a good choice; just keep in mind tandoori marinade usually contains yogurt, a lot of which is not very low-carb. Also, any kind of kabobs with meat and veggies are good as long as the meat is dry.

BBQ

Once of the biggest carb hang-ups, you'll come across at a BBQ joint is the sauces. Asking for your baby back ribs with no sauce does seem like it defeats the purpose. But BBQ restaurants are all about the smoking and the seasoning as well. A well-seasoned dry rubbed steak or rack of ribs will be just as enjoyable without the sauce. If asking for no sauce seems like a big deal you can always request it on the side. Sadly, just about every version of a BBQ sauce will be off limits due to the high amount of sugar, even in house-made sauces.

Also try to avoid pre-sauced dishes like pulled pork, barbacoa, or other shredded meats that are prepared in the sauce. Some southern BBQ places might use a sauce made with vinegar and mustard, which will be keto friendly.

If you're ordering wings, ask if there is a dry rub version (like they offer at Buffalo Wild Wings) or simply get them dry with buffalo sauce on the side. Pair them with ranch or blue cheese and celery sticks (try to avoid starchy carrots).

The same salad and side rules apply here as any other restaurant; steer clear of sweet, fruity dressings, hold the croutons, no bread or fried sides!

Sports Bars

Sports bars will probably have similar choices to chains like Applebee's, Chili's, and Buffalo Wild Wings, with the exception of limited nutrition facts and a few low carb choices on the menus. Still, the same concepts work for these non-chain restaurants.

If you're hanging with friends watching the big game, it's easy to just start munching on whatever lands on the table while you watch. Order all of your own appetizers and entrees rather than sharing orders with others who don't have the same diet requirements.

Steak is always a win, which will mostly likely be one of the options on the menu at a sports bar. The same goes for chicken, as long as it's not breaded. Grilled fish, pork chops, and bunless burgers are wise choices as well. Again, be mindful of sides and swap out dippable veggies like cucumbers and celery for the fries or potatoes.

Chapter 3: Keto Options at Convenience Stores & Gas Stations

Let's face it...we all need vacations in our lives! Figuring out what to eat once you're at your destination is one problem. What to eat along the way is another. Any long road trip or even time spent in an airport is going to require a pit stop of some kind. These stops are usually at stores with nothing but chips and candy...or so it seems. Even if there is no road trip involved, a quick trip to a 7/11 store to satisfy the "munchies" could be dangerous ground. Here are some quick, easy, and Keto friendly finds.

Cheese

Yes, cheese is our friend; and a very low-carb, fulfilling snack for on the go. You can get mozzarella string cheese or even jack or cheddar cheeses that come in a similar form. Make sure they are full fat and limit yourself to one or two to keep carbs down.

Raw Vegetables

Many convenience and gas station stores have small refrigerated sections where you can find great keto options, like raw veggies. Try to pick celery or broccoli over carrots and get a ranch dressing packet to go with it. Steer clear of peanut butter and hummus.

Hard Boiled Eggs

Perhaps not every convenience store will have these, but bigger ones like Walgreens or 7/11 might. These are the perfect keto snack and if the egg isn't enough you could even pair it with the veggies.

Cold Cuts

You might also find some cold cuts in the refrigerated section. Take care to read the ingredients, however. Some may be packed with sugary or really high sodium extras. These would also go well with the veggies and boiled eggs.

Jerky

Jerky is definitely an American staple! It is a great source of protein, and you can find it literally anywhere. Poultry jerkies will have less fat than beef, so go with the beef if you need to up your fat intake. Look at the ingredients before you buy it to make sure there aren't any added sugars and get original rather than flavored, like teriyaki.

Pork Rinds

These suckers have been around forever and have taken the keto world by storm! These are an excellent choice if you just need something to munch and you can even dip them in ranch or blue cheese if you need to.

Kale Chips

Kale chips are a fairly new addition to the convenience store roster and not every establishment will have them. If you find a store along the way that sells them, you might want to stock up for the rest of your trip. They are also an excellent substitute for chips or pretzels and can effectively satisfy the need to munch.

Hot Dogs

Any convenience store and most gas station stores will have a hot food section, with items like burritos, burgers, and hot dogs. The burgers will probably come already in the bun but the dogs are usually kept hot on their own. Grab one or two, skip the bun, add some mustard or ranch, and you have a Keto snack to go along with your veggies or kale chips.

Chapter 4: Keto Options: Low Carb Alcoholic & Coffee Beverages

For some, giving up alcohol or coffee may not be so bad. For others, it would be the end of the world! Have no fear; there are easily accessible low-carb options both at restaurants and coffee shops.

Keto Friendly Alcoholic Options

Wine & Beer: If you have to choose between one or the other, wines and champagnes have much fewer carbs than beer. Plus, beer is wheat based which will take your body out of ketosis very quickly.

For a keto diet, even if you're trying to stay below 20g net carbs a day, a glass of wine somewhat regularly would be alright. Try to choose dry wines as they will contain 0.5g sugar and under per glass. Definitely avoid ports and other sweet dessert wines. If there is not a suitable wine choice at the restaurant you might have to search for an alternative.

Beer is basically off limits period if you're trying to stay in ketosis unless you order very light American beers. But if you absolutely need a beer and the restaurant has very low carb choices, then you can safely have one *on occasion* if needed.

Spirits: Straight spirits are all 0g net carbs. It's the stuff that gets added to them you have to watch out for. For example, a vodka and soda water (aka "skinny bitch") is 0g net carbs while a Bloody Mary with vodka is 7g. When ordering mixed cocktails, avoid the ones with added sugars from syrups, sodas, and liqueurs. Dry martinis are also low-carb

Wine Coolers & Alcopops: all of these are off limits for keto diets. They are loaded with sugar; you're basically drinking a soda with some alcohol in it.

Keto Friendly Coffee Beverages

We all have that one friend who you would never want to meet in a dark alley on a caffeine rage. Or maybe you are that friend! Coffee is a staple for many to live through the day and it is very easy to find keto approved coffee beverages.

Starbucks Keto Drinks

Starbucks is probably the most well-known and widespread coffee chain in the world. They may not have too much going on for low-carb meals, but their keto coffee choices are quite vast and delicious.
Black Coffee: This one is kind of a no-brainer; if you want your coffee as low-carb as possibly, drink it black! Americanos are very low-carb as well.

Low-Carb Mocha: Replace the milk in the regular mocha with half water and half heavy cream. Ask for the skinny mocha sauce instead of regular.

Low-Carb Flat White: Replace steamed milk with half water, half heavy cream and you will maintain the creamy texture while cutting out much of the carbs.

Low-Carb Misto: Replace the milk with half and half water/heavy cream. Order it "short" and it will have only 5g net carbs (without modifications).

Low-Carb Vanilla Latte: Replace the milk with water/heavy cream and ask for sugar-free vanilla syrup.

Obviously, Starbucks is a coffee shop and can afford to be versatile. Ordering keto friendly coffee in fast food or sit down restaurants may be more difficult. When in doubt, always order it in black. If you have the option, get heavy cream instead of creamer. Or, you can bring your own MCT oil if it's the fatty taste you're craving.

Use the Starbucks guidelines for ordering espresso drinks at other establishments and beware of the syrups! If you have to have the syrup make sure it's always sugar free and you have substituted the milk for heavy cream.

Side note: all teas without honey or sugar are low carb, so knock yourself out!

Chapter 5: Keto Imposters & "Contraband"

If you feel like you have been sticking to the diet but are failing to see results, you may have been consuming "hidden" carbs and might have dropped out of ketosis.

Keto Imposters

There are the obvious slip-ups in sodas and candy. But even some reportedly healthy foods are not keto friendly at all. Cereals are some of the biggest imposters: 1 cup of cheerios has 17g net carbs, 1 cup of GoLean Crunch has 22g net carbs, Special K has 22g, and shredded wheat has a whopping 39g net carbs in a 1 cup serving!

Health or protein bars can also hide carbs. The chocolate chip Clif Bar alone has 41g net carbs! That's almost double the number of carbs in 1 serving that you should be eating in all your meals for one day on the keto diet.

Many Keto diet shopping lists include some fruits and nuts. In reality, most if not all should be avoided while trying to stay in ketosis. They are just too high in carbs to compensate for the fats and proteins they might be able to offer. The same goes for beans and legumes. If you have to have fruit in your life, choose low sugar berries such as blackberries, raspberries, or blueberries (try to keep serving sizes at ½ a cup or under).

Vegetables are definitely on the list, but not every vegetable is created equal. Take care limit and/or avoid starchy veggies such as sweet potatoes, regular potatoes, corn, carrots, peas, and even cherry tomatoes.

Sugars are an obvious no-no, but they often creep up even in foods we thought were healthy and keto friendly. Even "healthy" sugars can kick your body out of ketosis. Pay close attention to nutrition facts and try to avoid even natural sugars found in honey, syrups, raw sugar, agave nectar, and cane sugar.

Dairy is listed on Keto diets but still should be consumed in moderation and always full fat. Some dairy products that are not actually keto friendly are: low fat or 2% milks, low fat cottage cheese, pre-packaged shredded cheeses (which often include potato starch), low fat or substitute butters, and yogurts (both low and full fat as it is really hard to find low carb/sugar yogurts).

Keto Contraband

The keto diet could be described as fairly easy in, very easy out. In other words, it's not too difficult to go into ketosis (usually depending on what method you use) but it also doesn't take much to go out of it again. Part of making a lifestyle change includes kicking bad habits and cutting out bad foods...sometimes forever. The Keto diet may be temporarily based on your goals and health needs, and some foods may be "borderline" contraband. But if you're trying to remain in ketosis for any extended amount of time without having to start the process over, here are some foods to avoid at all costs in order to stay on track.

Some of the obvious ones that will kick your body out of ketosis are potatoes, all bread and grains (including pasta, even whole wheat), rice, beer, sodas, and juice, low fat dairy products, and yogurt.

Any coffee additives that are artificial (like creamers and sugars) should be avoided as well as cheese spread and some salad dressings. Many commercially made dressings, even potentially keto approved ones, have tons of added sugars. Steer clear of any fruit based dressings (such as berry vinaigrettes) and especially any labeled "low" or "reduced" fat; it's the fat you want, just not the carbs.

Most types of gravy and sauces are flour based to make them thicker and have added sugars for flavors. Finding any that are specifically low-carb at restaurants will be practically impossible, so it's best to always skip sauces and gravy when eating out if you want to stay in ketosis.

As we discussed earlier, there are a very few choices of fruit that are Keto friendly. Most of them should be avoided at all costs, due to their very high carb counts. These include Apples, kiwis, cherries, grapes, bananas, mangos, and citrus fruits.

Desserts that are sugary and/or bread and wheat based are also naturally off limits, such as candy and chocolate (unless it's at least 70% dark cacao), donuts, cakes, muffins, cupcakes, cake pops, and ice cream (unless it's specifically Keto friendly).

Chapter 6: Helpful Tips & Guidelines

One of the many perks of the Keto diet is, it has very few rules. There are so many foods you can eat (that taste great) and it fits perfectly into just about any exercise or training routine. That being said, there are some general easy-to-follow rules that will help you keep your body in ketosis when ordering food on the go.

Meats, Cheese, & Veggies

When in doubt, keep it simple! You won't always be able to quickly find pertinent nutrition facts at a restaurant, so sticking to these basics will keep you safe. Get your meat without sauces, especially if you can't find out if they have added sugars or not. Natural cheeses are preferable over American cheese, but either is fine. Ask for your veggies to be sautéed in butter if you don't like them steamed. Granted, this request may not fly at every dining spot, but many restaurants are happy to accommodate.

No Buns!

Bread is a sure way to carb load too much and knock your body out of ketosis. Even whole grains have a lot of sugar binding lectins in them. *If* you absolutely have to have bread and the restaurant can provide it, go with sprouted grains. But, the easiest option here is really to request the sandwich or burger wrapped in lettuce or served salad-style. Add-ons such as bacon or avocado will help satisfy you and ease the loss of the bread. Many sauces and condiments are keto appropriate; just make sure to keep an eye on the sugar content!

If ordering a salad (whether it started that way or you're creating your own) make sure to take into account *all* of the ingredients! Just because it's a salad, it doesn't mean you're always in the clear. Many salads come with croutons, nuts, or fruit, and high carb dressings. Even some leafy greens are higher in carbs. Go for salads that have meat in them to ensure you are getting enough fats and protein and when in doubt, get the dressing on the side. Greek restaurants are a good place to find delicious low-carb gyro-style salads. Skip all croutons and other carby/sugary ingredients and toppings.

Skip the Breading

The same concept for skipping buns goes for breading on fried foods as well if the breading is wheat based. If you really want what's underneath the breading, it's usually pretty easy to peel it off. You can then pair it with a fatty sauce like ranch or buffalo sauce. Or, you might even be able to order the dish without the breading (chicken wings, for example). There are keto-friendly breading options, such as crushed pork rinds, low-carb breadcrumbs, and parmesan and seasonings, but these types of breading will probably be difficult to impossible to find on a menu or even as a special request. It's always nice when the restaurant is accommodating, but we have to remember to not take it too far.

Watch Out for Condiments

Like we mentioned above, a vast majority of condiments and sauces are loaded with sugars and possibly even an overabundance of sodium (too much of a good thing and all that). Still, it is possible to use condiments and sauces to add flavor without getting into trouble. Any sweet-tasting sauces or dressings (like Teriyaki sauces or BBQ sauce) definitely have too much sugar for keto diets. Stick to fattier dressing and sauces like ranch (dressing or dip), buffalo sauce, sour cream (full fat), blue cheese, and Caesar. Keep in mind, some Caesar dressings are more sugary than others, so keep an eye on nutrition facts if possible. Plain yellow mustard is also a keto safe condiment and you could even ask for sides of butter if needed to get your daily fat intake up.

Making Special Requests

For some, the thought of being "that person" makes us squirm. But, at the end of the day, you have a responsibility to take care of yourself and as long as you keep requests respectful and attainable, you should have relatively little pushback. You should prepare yourself for some discomfort, but don't let that interfere with your health goals.

It's pretty standard these days to request burgers at fast food places without the bun; some joints even have these options on the main menu. Nutrition facts are also now readily available at any restaurant making it easier to quickly customize meal choices. You're more likely to get confused or irritated responses from employees for special requests made at fast food restaurants, so try to keep these as simple as possible. Asking for a burger "protein style" or lettuce wrapped is common enough. Don't give a long list of what you want or don't want; ask for cheese if you want cheese, specify toppings, then just get it dry. You can most likely get ranch and/or mustard easily enough on the side when you pick up your order. Be prepared for screw-ups on fast food special orders...it's just how it goes...and be grateful when they do get it right!

At sit down restaurants, you will be able to request more sophisticated alterations. It's actually pretty common to ask for no added salt to your meal and most sit down and family restaurants (chains especially) now have lite or low-carb sections in their menus. Those options make it much easier to get Keto appropriate meals without having to make special requests. Still, it is important to pay attention to additives listed in nutrition facts and sides that come with a meal. A grilled chicken dish is always a good low-carb choice. If it comes with steamed or even sautéed veggies, as long as butter or olive oil is used. However, these dishes are often served with rice, potatoes, and/or bread as well, which are definitely not Keto friendly. The a la carte options on menus could solve this problem well; you could always add a house salad to make the meal more complete. Keep in mind, however, this could also be a more expensive option. Chances are you could get the meal and opt out of those sides and even ask for double veggies to keep it filling.

Conclusion

Thanks for making it through to the end of *Keto Diet on the Go*, let's hope it was informative and able to provide you with all of the tools you need to achieve your goals whatever they may be.

The next step is to not be afraid to ask for low-carb options and to try new things. There are times when we fall into ruts when we start new routines because it's comfortable and easier to handle. Starting and sustaining a keto diet may not take as much discipline as other "fad" diets, but it will lose its appeal and ability to sustain if you let it get boring.

If you find yourself in a position where you have little to no info on the food you are ordering just follow the guidelines: meats, cheese, and vegetables. You can never go wrong with these keto basics and you can literally find them anywhere at any restaurant you go to.

A diet that revolves around fatty foods and still helps you lose weight is revolutionary. The more the world catches on to a healthier mind-set, we may see a rise in dining establishments providing low-carb options on their menus. So have fun with what you've learned and seize every opportunity for culinary adventure!

Finally, if you found this book useful in any way, a review on Amazon is always appreciated!

Made in the USA
San Bernardino, CA
18 May 2019